The Ultimate Fertility Diet Cookbook: Boost Your Chances of Conceiving with Delicious Recipe

By

Joyce Lifted

COPYRIGHT

All rights reserved. No part of this publication may be republished in any form or by any means, including translation, scanning, photocopying, etc., without the prior written permission of the copyright owner.

TABLE OF CONTENTS

Fertility treatment introduction 1

Building block of a fertility diet.........................2

Meal Planning for Fertility 3

Breakfasts for Fertility **4**

Snacks and Appetizers for Fertility 5

Soups and Salads for Fertility 6

Healthy diet for ovulation boost...........................**7**

Main Dishes for Fertility 8

Sides and Vegetables for Fertility....................9

Desserts for Fertility **10**

Beverages for Fertility.................................11

Fertility-Boosting Ingredients 12

Meal Planning for Special Diets **13**

Chapter 1

Fertility Treatment Introduction

This book is an overview of how diet affects fertility, including tips on creating a nutritional plan to boost fertility.

Fertility is an important aspect of human life and many couples suffer from infertility. Diet has been shown to play an important role in improving or affecting the foods you eat. This can affect hormone balance, ovulation, sperm quality, and overall reproductive health.

Having a fertility-enhancing meal plan is an important step in increasing your chances of conceiving. A fertility diet is an eating plan that focuses on avoiding foods that can affect fertility and consuming foods that have been shown to increase fertility.

Foods included in fertility treatments are as follows;

Plant Foods

Eating plant-based foods such as fruits, vegetables, nuts, and whole grains is essential to boost fertility. These foods provide antioxidants that help regulate hormone levels and improve egg quality that is rich in substances, fiber, and other essential nutrients.

Healthy Fats

Eating healthy fats, such as the omega-3 fatty acids found in fish, chia seeds and flaxseeds can help reduce inflammation and promote ovulation.

Protein

Eating high-protein foods such as red meat, beans and lentils can help regulate insulin levels and improve egg quality. Low glycemic index foods:

Eating foods with a low glycemic index, such as sweet potatoes, quinoa, and lentils, can help regulate insulin levels and improve fertility.

FOODS TO AVOID DURING FERTILITY TREATMENT

Here are few food to avoid when trying conceive or during fertility treatment.

1. Trans Fat: Eating Trans fats are found in fast food, fried foods, and processed snacks, can increase insulin resistance and reduce fertility.
2. Food with A High Glycemic Index: Eating foods with a high glycemic index, such as white bread, pasta, and rice, can cause insulin spikes and reduce fertility.
3. Alcohol and Caffeine: Alcohol and caffeine consumption can affect fertility, so it's best to limit or avoid your intake of these substances.

Chapter 2

Building Blocks of a Fertility Diet

When trying to conceive, many couples resort to fertility treatments and medications to increase their chances of conceiving. But an often overlooked aspect of fertility is the role nutrition plays in improving reproductive health. Fertility treatment involves consuming certain foods and nutrients that can support reproductive health and increase the chances of conception.

A fertility diet focuses on nutrient-dense whole foods that provide an array of vitamins, minerals and antioxidants that are important for reproductive health. It includes a combination of foods, healthy fats, lean protein, complex carbohydrates, iron-rich foods, and water. Plant-based foods are an essential component of a fertility diet. Eating a variety of colorful fruits and vegetables provides important nutrients such as folic acid, vitamin C and antioxidants, which may improve fertility. For example, folic acid is essential for healthy fetal development. And may help reduce the risk of not been able to put to birth. Vitamin C can improve sperm quality and increase the chances of conception. Antioxidants such as beta-carotene and lycopene help prevent oxidation it can protect against stress and improve egg quality. Aim to eat at least five servings of fruits and vegetables a day, and include leafy greens, berries, citrus fruits, and cruciferous vegetables such as broccoli and cauliflower.

Healthy fats are also important for fertility. Omega-3 fatty acids found in foods such as salmon, nuts and seeds help regulate hormones and improve ovulation. Monounsaturated and polyunsaturated fats found in olive oil, avocados, and nuts are also beneficial. These healthy fats help balance hormone levels and reduce inflammation in the body. Incorporating healthy fats into your diet can support healthy ovulation and increase your chances of conception.

Lean protein such as chicken, fish and beans is another important component of fertility treatment. Eating lean protein provides essential amino acids for reproductive health. Amino acids are the building blocks of proteins and are important for cell function and tissue repair. It also helps regulate hormone levels and promotes healthy egg and sperm development. Be sure to include a variety of protein sources in your diet, including plant-based options like lentils and chickpeas.

Complex carbohydrates are also important for fertility. Opt for whole grains like quinoa, brown rice, and oats instead of refined crabs like white bread and pasta. They help regulate blood sugar and insulin levels, which are important for fertility. High insulin levels can interfere with ovulation and increase the risk of conditions such as polycystic ovary syndrome (PCOS). I have. Complex carbohydrates can also provide fiber, which helps regulate digestion and reduce inflammation in the body.

Iron-rich foods are important for fertility because iron is an important nutrient for reproductive health. Iron is important for the production of healthy red blood cells, which carry oxygen to body tissues. Iron is also important for healthy egg and sperm development. Iron is found in foods such as red meat, spinach, and lentils. If you are iron deficient, your doctor may recommend iron supplements.

Water is an essential part of fertility treatment. Staying hydrated is important for our overall health, including reproductive health. You should aspire to drink at least 8 cups of water daily. Be sure to drink more water if you are exercising or in hot weather. Staying hydrated is important when trying to conceive, as dehydration can impair the production of healthy cervical mucus and reduce sperm motility. It's important to remember that fertility treatment is only one aspect of improving reproductive health. Other lifestyle factors such as exercise, stress management, and adequate sleep are also important. Regular exercise improves circulation and reduces stress.

Chapter 3

Meal Planning for Fertility

Meal planning is an essential part of staying healthy, and this is especially true for those trying to conceive. Eating a balanced diet that supports reproductive health can increase your chances of conceiving Increase. A fertility diet plan is all about making sure you're eating the right foods in the right amounts to support reproductive health. Here are some helpful tips.

Focus On Natural Foods

Whole foods are foods that are minimally processed and provide a range of essential vitamins and minerals. These foods are nutrient dense and rich in nutrients per calorie. Examples of whole foods are fresh fruits, vegetables, whole grains, lean proteins and healthy fats. Incorporating these foods into your diet will ensure that you are getting the essential nutrients you need for reproductive health.

Incorporate Foods That Support Hormonal Balance

Hormonal imbalance can lead to irregular ovulation and reduced fertility. Eating foods that support hormonal balance can help improve reproductive health. Foods high in omega-3 fatty acids, such as salmon and flaxseed, help regulate hormones. Leafy greens such as spinach and kale help regulate estrogen levels. Incorporating these foods into your diet can help support hormonal balance and increase your chances of getting pregnant.

Add Essential Nutrients

Certain nutrients such as folic acid, iron and zinc are essential for fertility. Make sure foods rich in these nutrients are included in your diet. Examples of foods high in folic acid include spinach, lentils, and nuts. Foods rich in iron include lean red meats and dark leafy vegetables. Oyster and pumpkin seeds are excellent sources of zinc.

Focus On Complex Carbohydrates

Complex carbohydrates are essential for maintaining healthy blood sugar levels. High blood sugar can lead to insulin resistance, which can affect ovulation and reduce fertility. Examples of complex carbohydrates are whole grains, starchy vegetables, and legumes. Avoid refined carbohydrates, such as white bread and pasta, which can cause blood sugar spikes.

Drink Enough

Drinking enough water throughout the day is important for overall health, including reproductive health. Drinking water keeps your body hydrated and supports reproductive health. If you find it difficult to drink plain water, try adding fruit and herbs to add flavor.

Planning meal When you're on the go all the time, it is not easy to make healthy food choices. By planning ahead, you can avoid making unhealthy choices. Our pre-cut fruits, veggies, nuts and healthy granola bars are great for healthy on-the-go snacks.

In summary, dietary planning for fertility is about including the right foods in your diet to support reproductive health. Whole foods, foods that support hormonal balance, essential nutrients, and complex carbohydrates, are an important part of any fertility-friendly diet plan. Stay hydrated and plan ahead for healthy meals and snacks to stick to your meal plan. Making these changes to your diet and meal plan can increase your chances of getting pregnant and improve your overall health.

Chapter 4

Breakfasts for Fertility

Starting the day off with a healthy breakfast is important for everyone, but it is especially important for those who are trying to conceive. A balanced breakfast can provide the necessary nutrients to support reproductive health and increase the chances of getting pregnant. In this chapter, we will explore some of the best breakfast options for improving fertility.

Smoothie Bowls

Smoothie bowls are a great way to pack a lot of nutrients into one meal. They are typically made with a blend of fruits and vegetables, which provide a range of essential vitamins and minerals. Adding protein-rich ingredients like nut butter or Greek yogurt can help to keep you feeling full and satisfied until lunchtime.

Oatmeal

Oatmeal is a classic breakfast option that is rich in fiber and complex carbohydrates. This slow-burning energy source can help to regulate blood sugar levels, which is important for reproductive health. Adding fruits, nuts, or seeds to your oatmeal can help to increase the nutrient density of your meal.

Eggs

Eggs are an excellent source of protein, which is essential for reproductive health. They also contain chorine, which is important for fetal brain development. Enjoying a veggie omelet or a boiled egg with whole grain toast can be a great way to start the day.

Greek Yogurt

Greek yogurt is high in protein and contains probiotics that can help support a healthy gut. Adding fruits or nuts to your yogurt can increase the nutrient density of your meal. Look for plain Greek yogurt, as flavored varieties can be high in added sugar.

Avocado Toast

Avocado toast has become a popular breakfast option in recent years, and for good reason. Avocados are a great source of healthy fats and fiber, which can help to regulate blood sugar levels. Top your avocado toast with a boiled egg or some smoked salmon for an extra protein boost.

Quinoa Breakfast Bowl

Quinoa is a nutrient-dense grain that is high in protein and fiber. Making a breakfast bowl with quinoa, fruits, nuts, and seeds can be a great way to start the day. Add some Greek yogurt or a drizzle of honey for some added sweetness.

Berry Parfait

Berries are high in antioxidants, which can help to support reproductive health. Layering berries, Greek yogurt, and granola can be a delicious and nutritious way to start the day. Look for low-sugar granola or make your own to avoid added sugars.

Chia Pudding

Chia seeds are high in omega-3 fatty acids and fiber, which can help to support reproductive health. Making a chia pudding with almond milk berries, and nuts can be a delicious and healthy breakfast option. You can also add a touch of honey or maple syrup for some added sweetness.

In conclusion, a healthy breakfast is an essential part of meal planning for fertility. Incorporating nutrient-dense foods like fruits, vegetables, whole grains, lean proteins, and healthy fats into your breakfast can help to support reproductive health and increase your chances of getting pregnant. Smoothie bowls, oatmeal, eggs, Greek yogurt, avocado toast, quinoa breakfast bowls, berry parfaits, and chia pudding are all great options for a fertility-friendly breakfast. By making these changes to your diet, you can improve your chances of getting pregnant and support your overall health.

Chapter 5

Snacks and Appetizers for Fertility

Fertility is a complex and multifaceted aspect of human health that can be influenced by various factors such as genetics, age, lifestyle choices, and diet. While there is no one-size-fits-all approach to promoting fertility, certain nutrients and foods have been shown to support reproductive health in both men and women.

When it comes to snacking and appetizers, it is important to choose foods that are not only tasty but also provide a good balance of nutrients that support fertility. In this article, we will explore some of the best snacks and appetizers for fertility.

Nuts and Seeds

Nuts and seeds are a good source of healthy fats, fiber, and protein. They are also rich in antioxidants and other nutrients that support fertility such as zinc, selenium, and vitamin E.

Some of the best nuts and seeds for fertility include almonds, walnuts, pumpkin seeds, and sesame seeds.

Avocado

Avocado is a nutrient-dense fruit that is rich in healthy fats, fiber, and vitamins such as vitamin E and foliate. It also contains a variety of antioxidants that can help to protect reproductive cells from oxidative stress. Avocado can be enjoyed on its own, as a dip, or as a spread on toast.

Berries

Berries such as strawberries, blueberries, and raspberries are packed with antioxidants, vitamins, and minerals that support fertility. They are also low in calories and high in fiber, making them a great snack option for those looking to maintain a healthy weight.

Greek Yogurt

Greek yogurt is a great source of protein and calcium, both of which are essential for reproductive health. It also contains probiotics, which can help to support gut health and improve nutrient absorption. Greek yogurt can be enjoyed on its own or as a base for dips and spreads.

Hummus

Hummus is a delicious dip made from chickpeas, and other ingredients. It is a great source of protein, fiber, and healthy fats, as well as a variety of vitamins and minerals such as iron, magnesium, and foliates. Hummus can be enjoyed with vegetables, crackers, or as a spread on sandwiches.

Dark Chocolate

Dark chocolate is a delicious and nutritious snack that is rich in antioxidants and other nutrients that support fertility. It is also a natural mood booster, which can help to reduce stress and anxiety. Dark chocolate can be enjoyed on its own or as a topping for fruits and nuts.

Edamame

Edamame is a type of soybean that is rich in protein, fiber, and a variety of vitamins and minerals such as iron and calcium. It is also a good source of phytoestrogens, which can help to balance hormones and improve reproductive health. Edamame can be enjoyed on its own, as a snack, or as an ingredient in salads and stir-fries.

Hard-Boiled Eggs

Eggs are a great source of protein, healthy fats, and a variety of vitamins and minerals that support fertility. Hard-boiled eggs are a convenient and easy snack option that can be enjoyed on their own or as a topping for salads and sandwiches.

Sweet Potato

Sweet potatoes are delicious and nutritious snack that are rich in fiber, vitamins, and minerals such as beta-carotene and potassium. They are also a good source of complex carbohydrates, which can help to regulate blood sugar and support reproductive health. Sweet potatoes can be enjoyed on their own or as a base for dips and spreads.

In conclusion, snacking and appetizers can be a great way to support fertility by providing a good balance of nutrients that promote reproductive health. By incorporating these foods into your diet, you can help to support your overall health and increase your chances of conceiving. However, it's important to keep in mind that while diet can play a role in fertility, it's not the only factor. Other lifestyle choices such as exercise, stress management, and avoiding smoking and excessive alcohol consumption also play an important role.

When it comes to fertility, it's also important to seek the advice of a healthcare professional. If you are struggling to conceive, a doctor or a fertility specialist can help you to identify potential underlying issues and provide you with treatment options.

Finally, it's worth noting that these snack and appetizer suggestions are not just beneficial for those trying to conceive. They are nutritious and healthy options that can benefit anyone, regardless of their reproductive goals. By incorporating a variety of these foods into your diet, you can help to support your overall health and wellbeing.

Chapter 6

Soups and Salads for Fertility

Maintaining good reproductive health is important for couples who want to conceive. Fertility depends on many factors, including genetics and age, but lifestyle choices such as diet also play an important role in supporting reproductive health. Eating a balanced diet containing foods rich in key nutrients can help improve fertility and increase your chances of conception. Soups and salads provide a wide range of nutrients to support fertility. Two excellent meals you can have.

Fertility soup

Soup is a comforting, nutritious meal that can be easily adapted to contain a variety of ingredients that are beneficial to fertility. Here are some soups that you might want to include in your diet.

Vegetable Soup

Vegetable soups are great for those looking to increase their intake of fertility-supporting vitamins and minerals. This soup contains a variety of vegetables rich in vitamins A, C, E and folic acid, including carrots, sweet potatoes, kale, and spinach. Can be made with

Lentil soup

Lentil soup is a great source of plant-based protein and fiber that supports reproductive health. Lentils are also high in iron, an essential nutrient for women trying to conceive.

Chicken Soup

Chicken soup is a traditional comfort food that can provide an array of nutrients that support fertility. Chicken is an excellent source of lean protein, and vegetables such as carrots and celery provide an array of vitamins and minerals that are beneficial to reproductive health.

Salad for Fertility

Salads are a great option for those looking to increase their intake of nutrient-packed fruits and vegetables that support fertility.

Spinach and strawberry salad

Spinach and strawberries are both rich in vitamin C and can help improve sperm and egg quality. This salad should be topped with nuts and seeds, which are great sources of healthy fats and protein.

Kale quinoa salad

Kale is a super food packed with an array of nutrients that support fertility, including vitamins A, C, and K. Quinoa is an excellent source of vegetable protein and fiber, and is also rich in iron.

Avocado and tomato salad

Avocados are a great source of healthy fats, and tomatoes are rich in lycopene, which helps improve sperm quality. This salad is made with olive oil and vinegar, both sources of healthy fats.

You can dress it up with the simple vinaigrette you made.

Other Fertility Boosting Ingredients

In addition to the soups and salads above, there are several other ingredients you may want to incorporate into your diet to support fertility.

Leafy vegetables

Leafy greens like spinach, kale, and chard provide a range of nutrients that support reproductive health. This vegetable is rich in folic acid and vitamins A, C and K that are essential for fetal development.

Nuts and seeds

Nuts and seeds are not only great sources of healthy fats, proteins and fiber. They also contain a variety of vitamins and minerals that support fertility. Walnuts, almonds and sunflower seeds are great choices.

Fruits

Fruits such as oranges, strawberries, and blueberries are rich in vitamin C, which helps improve sperm and egg quality. It's also a great source of antioxidants that help protect germ cells from damage. In summary, a balanced diet containing soups and salads rich in essential nutrients can help improve fertility and increase your chances of conception.

Chapter 7

Healthy diet for ovulation boost

Healthy ovulation is a key component of reproductive health and plays an essential role in pregnancy. If you're trying to conceive, it's important to understand how your diet supports ovulation and increases your chances of getting pregnant. This chapter explores nutrition to promote healthy ovulation, including nutrients you need, foods to eat (and avoid), recipes to support healthy ovulation, and strategies for creating fertility plan.

Nutrients needed for ovulation

Ovulation is a complex process that requires the coordination of several hormones, including estrogen, progesterone, follicle-stimulating hormone (FSH), and luteinizing hormone (LH). These hormones work together to stimulate the growth and release of eggs from the ovaries, which can be fertilized by sperm. To support healthy ovulation, your body needs a variety of nutrients including iron, folic acid, vitamin D and omega-3 fatty acids. Iron is important in the formation of hemoglobin, which carries oxygen to the body's cells, including the ovaries. Folic acid is important for cell division and DNA synthesis, especially during early pregnancy. Vitamin D is necessary for bone health, immune function, hormone regulation, and has been associated with improved fertility. Omega-3 fatty acids have anti-inflammatory properties and have been shown to improve ovulation and increase the chances of conception.

Foods That Promote Healthy Ovulation to get the nutrients you need for healthy ovulation, it's important to eat a balanced diet rich in fruits and vegetables, lean protein, healthy fats and whole grains.

Leafy vegetables:

Spinach, kale, and other leafy greens are rich sources of iron, folic acid, and other important nutrients. They are also a great source of antioxidants that can protect the ovaries from damage.

Fatty fish:

Salmon, tuna, and other fatty fish are rich in omega-3 fatty acids that help regulate hormones and improve ovulation. It is also a good source of vitamin D. ## Nuts and Seeds:

Almonds, walnuts, chia seeds and flaxseeds are rich in healthy fats and protein and are also good sources of vitamins and minerals such as vitamin E, zinc and magnesium.

Full grain:

Brown rice, quinoa, and other whole grains are rich in fiber, which helps regulate hormones and improve ovulation. It is also an excellent source of B vitamins, which are important for energy and hormone regulation.

On the other hand, certain foods can interfere with ovulation and reduce your chances of getting pregnant. It is best to limit or avoid processed foods, Tran's fats, and excessive caffeine and alcohol. If you're looking for recipe ideas to support healthy ovulation, consider these options.

Smoothies

Mix spinach, almond milk, frozen berries and chia seeds together for a hearty breakfast rich in iron, antioxidants and omega-3 fatty acids.

Salad

Toss your salad with spinach, grilled salmon, walnuts and avocado for a meal rich in protein, healthy fats and vitamins.

Main course:

Try the quinoa bowl with roasted sweet potatoes, black beans and avocado.

Snack:

Spread almond butter on apple slices or whole wheat crackers for a snack rich in protein, healthy fats and fiber.

Creating a fertility treatment plan

A fertility nutrition plan is important to ensure you get the nutrients you need for healthy ovulation.

Chapter 8

Main Dishes for Fertility

Infertility is a problem that has become more and more important in recent years as more and more couples struggle to conceive. There are many factors that affect fertility, including genetics, age, and lifestyle. Also play an important role. In this chapter, we examine some main dishes that have been shown to increase fertility.

Grilled salmon with quinoa salad

Salmon is a good source of protein, omega-3 fatty acids and vitamin D, all of which help improve fertility. Quinoa, on the other hand, is a complex carbohydrate rich in fiber, protein, and other essential nutrients. It has a low glycemic index.

For this dish, he marinates the salmon fillets in olive oil, lemon juice, and herbs of your choice for over 30 minutes. Then grill the salmon. Serve with a quinoa salad made with diced vegetables such as cucumbers, red onions, and bell peppers, and lemon vinaigrette. Stir-fried vegetables with brown rice

A diet rich in vegetables has been shown to improve fertility in both men and women. Vegetables are rich in antioxidants, which protect eggs and sperm from free radical damage. It is also a good source of vitamins and minerals such as vitamin C, folic acid and iron, which are important for reproductive health.

To prepare this dish, various vegetables such as broccoli, carrots, green peppers and snow peas are sautéed in a little oil. Season with garlic and ginger, then soy sauce or tamari. Serve vegetables over brown rice, a complex carbohydrate high in fiber and low in glycemic index.

Lentil Soup with Whole Grain Bread

Lentils are a great source of plant-based protein, fiber and iron, all of which help improve fertility. Iron is important for women who want to conceive. A lack of iron can lead to anemia, which can make it difficult to conceive. Whole grain bread is another good source of complex carbohydrates and fiber.

For this dish, onions, garlic and carrots are sautéed in a little oil until soft. Add dried lentils, vegetable stock, and your favorite herbs and spices. Bring the soup to a boil, then reduce the heat and simmer until the lentils are tender. Serve the soup with whole grain bread.

Beef and vegetable stew

Beef is an excellent source of protein and iron, both of which are important for fertility. Iron is important for the production of hemoglobin, which carries oxygen to the reproductive organs. Vegetables such as carrots, potatoes and onions are also rich in essential nutrients and antioxidants.

In this dish, beef he cubes are fried in a small amount of oil. Add the diced vegetables and your favorite herbs and spices and pour over the beef broth. Simmer the stew until the beef is tender and the vegetables are cooked through. Serve the stew with whole grain bread. Chickpea curry with basmati rice

Chickpeas are an excellent source of vegetable protein, fiber and iron. It also contains a lot of folic acid, which is important for women trying to conceive. Basmati rice is a low-glycemic carbohydrate, high in fiber and has a nutty flavor.

Chapter 9

Sides and Vegetables for Fertility

A balanced and nutritious diet is important to improve fertility. While the main course provides most of the nutrients, side dishes and vegetables are equally important in providing essential vitamins and minerals that support reproductive health.

Roasted sweet potato

Sweet potatoes are an excellent source of vitamin A, which is important for reproductive health in both men and women. Vitamin A is essential for healthy sperm and egg cell development. To prepare this food, you have to preheat your oven to 400°F. Dice the sweet potato and toss with olive oil, salt and pepper. Roast in oven for 25 to 30 minutes or until tender and golden brown.

Broccoli with garlic and lemon

Broccoli is rich in folic acid, a B vitamin important for reproductive health. Folic acid is necessary for DNA synthesis and cell division, and a deficiency can lead to birth defects and infertility. Garlic is also beneficial for fertility as it contains selenium which is important for sperm health.

In this dish, the broccoli is steamed until light green and tender. While the broccoli is cooking, fry the garlic in a little oil until fragrant. Mix garlic with boiled broccoli and sprinkle with lemon juice.

Grilled Brussels sprouts

Brussels sprouts are an excellent source of vitamin C, which is important for reproductive health. Vitamin C is an antioxidant that protects sperm and egg cells from free radical damage. Brussels sprouts are also rich in folic acid and fiber.

To prepare this dish, preheat your oven to 400°F. Cut the Brussels sprouts in half and mix with olive oil, salt and pepper. Roast in oven for 25-30 minutes or until tender and golden brown. Spinach salad with berries and nuts

Spinach is rich in iron, which is important for reproductive health. Iron is required for the production of hemoglobin, which carries oxygen to the reproductive organs. Berries are rich in antioxidants that protect sperm and egg cells from damage. Nuts are rich in healthy fats that are important for hormone production.

For this dish, spinach leaves are mixed with sliced strawberries, blueberries and chopped nuts. Drizzle with balsamic vinegar.

Roasted asparagus

Asparagus is an excellent source of vitamin E, which is important for male fertility. Vitamin E is an antioxidant that protects sperm from damage.

Asparagus is also rich in folic acid and dietary fiber.

To prepare this dish, he preheats the oven to 400°F. Cut off the tips of the asparagus and toss with olive oil, salt and pepper. Roast in the oven for 10 to 15 minutes or until tender and lightly browned.

In summary, incorporating nutrient-rich side dishes and vegetables into your diet can support fertility. Sweet potatoes, broccoli, Brussels sprouts, spinach, and asparagus are just a few examples of foods rich in vitamins and minerals essential for reproductive health. Additionally, it's important to aim for a balanced and varied diet that includes a variety of whole foods and minimizes processed and high-fat foods.

Chapter 10

Desserts for Fertility

The idea of using desserts to boost fertility may seem far-fetched, but there are certain foods that have been shown to improve reproductive health in both men and women. Let's take a look at some of these foods and how they can be incorporated into delicious and nutritious desserts.

First of all, it is important to note that fertility is influenced by many factors, including age, genetics, lifestyle choices, and underlying medical conditions. Diet alone cannot guarantee fertility, but it certainly plays a role in optimizing reproductive health. In fact, a study published in the journal Fertility and Sterility found that women who followed a Mediterranean diet high in fruits, vegetables, whole grains, and lean protein were more likely to conceive through in vitro fertilization (IVF). It turns out those Women who did not follow this type of diet. Antioxidants are an important part of a fertility-enhancing diet.

Antioxidants are compounds in food that protect cells from damage caused by free radicals, unstable molecules that can damage DNA and other cellular components. Related to fertility, antioxidants have been shown to improve sperm quality in men and reduce oxidative stress in women, which may improve the chances of ovulation and conception.

The best sources of antioxidants include berries, citrus fruits, nuts and dark chocolate. These foods can be incorporated into a variety of desserts such as: B. Fruit salads, smoothies, and chocolate-based treats. For example, a simple yet delicious dessert is a mixed berry salad with chopped nuts and a drizzle of dark chocolate sauce.

Another nutrient important to fertility is omega-3 fatty acids. Omega-3 fatty acids are a class of polyunsaturated fatty acids that are important for brain and heart health and reduce inflammation in the body. Regarding fertility, omega-3 fatty acids have been shown to improve sperm quality, regulate the menstrual cycle, and improve implantation chances in women undergoing in vitro fertilization.

Some of the best sources of omega-3 fatty acids are fatty fish such as salmon, sardines and mackerel, and nuts and seeds such as walnuts, flaxseeds and chia seeds. These foods can be incorporated into desserts in creative ways such as: Examples include using ground flaxseeds or chia seeds as part of the flour in baked goods, or adding chopped nuts or salmon to quinoa-based desserts.

In addition to antioxidants and omega-3 fatty acids, there are certain vitamins and minerals that are important for fertility. For example, folic acid, a type of B vitamin, is important for the fetal development and reduces the risk of birth defects. Zinc, a mineral found in meat, seafood and nuts, is important for sperm production and has been shown to improve male fertility.

An easy way to incorporate these nutrients into your desserts is to make smoothies and shakes that are fortified with vitamins and minerals. For example, a banana and avocado smoothie can be made with almond milk and fortified with folic acid and zinc supplements. The idea is to create a yogurt-based dessert topped with chopped nuts and fresh fruit.

In conclusion, dessert alone cannot guarantee fertility, but including certain foods and nutrients in desserts can be a delicious and nutritious way to support reproductive health. By focusing on foods rich in antioxidants, omega-3 fatty acids, vitamins and minerals, you can create delicious and fertility-friendly desserts. Whether you're trying to conceive or looking for ways to optimize your health, these desserts are sure to satisfy your sweet tooth.

Chapter 11

Beverages for Fertility

Beverages are an integral part of our daily lives and also play a role in enhancing fertility. This chapter reviews some of the beverages that have been shown to improve reproductive health in both men and women.

Water is probably the most important drink for fertility. Staying hydrated is very important for overall health and especially important for reproductive health. Dehydration can lead to decreased cervical mucus, which can make it harder for sperm to reach the egg. It can also affect the thickness of the endometrial, which can make implantation of a fertilized egg more difficult.

In addition to water, there are certain beverages that may further increase fertility. One of the most popular fertility drinks is green tea. Green tea is a type of tea made from unfermented leaves and is high in antioxidants called catechins. Catechins have been shown to improve sperm quality and reduce oxidative stress in women. This may improve the chances of ovulation and conception. A study published in the journal Fertility and Sterility found that women who drank green tea were more likely to become pregnant through in vitro fertilization than those who did not. Another study published in the American Journal of Clinical Nutrition found that men who consumed more green tea had higher sperm concentration and motility than men who did not consume green tea.

In addition to green tea, there are other herbal teas that are useful in treating fertility. For example, red raspberry leaf tea is a popular herbal tea thought to improve uterine health and tone uterine muscles. Not only does this make it easier for the uterus to contract during labor, but it also helps regulate the menstrual cycle and improve fertility. Another herbal tea often recommended for fertility treatment is nettle tea. Made from nettle leaves, nettle tea is rich in vitamins and minerals that are important for reproductive health. For example, nettle tea is a good source of iron, which is important for healthy circulation and the prevention of anemia. It is also a good source of calcium, which is important for strong bones and teeth.

In addition to tea, there are certain juices that are beneficial for fertility. One of the most popular fertility juices is pomegranate juice. Pomegranate juice is rich in antioxidants and has been shown to improve sperm quality in men. It has also been shown to reduce oxidative stress in women and increase the chances of ovulation and conception.

Another juice often recommended for fertility is beet juice. Beet juice is high in nitrates and improves blood flow and oxygen supply to the uterus and ovaries. Beet juice is also a good source of folate, which is important for fetal development and has been shown to reduce the risk of birth defects.

In addition to teas and juices, there are certain alcoholic beverages that can moderately help with fertility. An example is red wine. Red wine is high in an antioxidant called resveratrol, which has been shown to improve sperm quality in men and reduce oxidative stress in women. However, it's important to note that excessive alcohol consumption can adversely affect fertility and overall health.

Finally, it's important to mention the role caffeine plays in fertility. Caffeine is a stimulant found in coffee, tea, chocolate, and more.

Chapter 12

Fertility-Boosting Ingredients

Fertility-enhancing ingredients are those that have been shown to improve reproductive health in both men and women. Check whether to

Omega 3 fatty acids

Omega-3 fatty acids are a type of healthy fat found in certain foods such as fatty fish, nuts and seeds. It has been shown to improve sperm quality in men and regulate ovulation in women. Omega-3 fatty acids also help reduce inflammation in the body and can improve overall reproductive health.

Zinc

Zinc is an essential mineral important for many bodily functions, including reproductive health. It plays an important role in sperm production and helps regulate the menstrual cycle in women. Zinc is also important for healthy acolyte and embryo development. Foods rich in zinc include oysters, beef, and pumpkin seeds.

Folic acid

Folic acid is a B vitamin that is important for fetal development and helps prevent birth defects. It's also important for women trying to conceive because it helps regulate ovulation and increase the chances of conception. Foods high in folic acid include green leafy vegetables, citrus fruits, and beans.

Vitamin D

Vitamin D is an essential vitamin important for bone health and immune function. It has also been shown to be involved in reproductive health. Vitamin D deficiency is associated with infertility in both men and women, and vitamin D supplementation has been shown to improve fertility. Foods rich in vitamin D include fatty fish, egg yolks, and fortified dairy products.

Selenium

Selenium is an essential mineral important for many bodily functions, including reproductive health. Plays an important role in sperm production and helps protect the testicles from damage. Selenium has also been shown to reduce the risk of miscarriage and increase the chances of conception. Selenium-rich foods Brazil nuts, tuna, and turkey. L-arginine

L-Arginine is an amino acid that is important for many bodily functions, including reproductive health. It plays an important role in sperm production and helps improve sperm quality and motility. L-Arginine has also been shown to improve blood flow to the reproductive organs. This may improve overall fertility. Foods rich in L-arginine include turkey, chicken, and pumpkin seeds.

Coenzyme Q10

Coenzyme Q10 is a powerful antioxidant important for many bodily functions, including reproductive health. Plays an important role in energy production and helps protect eggs and sperm from damage. Coenzyme Q10 has also been shown to improve egg quality in women over the age of 35. Rich in Coenzyme Q10 Foods include fatty fish, offal, and peanuts.

Maca root

Maca root is a type of plant native to Peru. It has been used for centuries as a natural remedy for infertility and hormonal imbalances. Maca root is rich in nutrients important for reproductive health, including iron, zinc and vitamin C. It has also been shown to improve sperm count and motility in men, regulate the menstrual cycle, and improve fertility in women.

Ashwagandha

Ashwagandha is an herb native to India. It has been used for centuries as a natural remedy for infertility and hormonal imbalances. Ashwagandha is rich in antioxidants and helps protect eggs and sperm from damage. It has also been shown to improve sperm count and motility in men, regulate the menstrual cycle, and improve fertility.

Chapter 13

Meal Planning for Special Diets

Meal planning can be difficult for everyone, but it can be especially difficult for those on special diets. Can make it more difficult to find recipes and plan meals. This chapter reviews some tips for planning meals for special diets.

Identify nutritional needs

The first step in planning a special diet is determining your nutritional needs. These can be allergies, intolerances, ailments, or personal preferences. Once you know what to avoid and what to include in your diet, you can search for recipes and plan your meals accordingly.

Research recipe

The internet is a great resource for finding recipes for special meals. There are many blogs and websites that focus on specific diets such as gluten-free, dairy-free, vegan, etc. You can also use search engines to find recipes that meet your dietary needs. Read the recipe carefully to make sure it meets your dietary needs. Plan a meal

Once you have your list of recipes, you can start planning your meals. This includes planning meals for the week and creating meal plans for the entire month. Consider special events or occasions that require a different meal plan.

Make a shopping list

After creating a meal plan, you can create a shopping list. This keeps you organized and ensures that you have all the ingredients you need for your meal. Check the ingredients to make sure they meet your dietary needs.

Prepare in advance

Meal prep is a great way to save time and always have healthy meals on hand. This may include prior material preparation such as: B. Cut vegetables or cook grains. You can also prepare a full meal in advance and store it in the freezer for later.

Be creative

Following a special diet does not mean you have to eat the same thing every day. Be creative and try new recipes. You can also experiment with different herbs and spices to add flavor to your dishes.

Focus on natural foods

Regardless of your dietary needs, it's important to focus on whole foods. That means eating foods that are as close to their natural state as possible: fruits, vegetables, whole grains, lean proteins, etc. Whole foods are more nutritious and can help improve your overall health. Read the label carefully

When buying groceries, read the labels carefully. This will help you identify potentially problematic ingredients in your diet. If you are unsure about any ingredient, do your research or consult your doctor.

Use alternatives

If you're on a special diet, they often substitute for common ingredients. For example, if you are lactose intolerant, you can substitute almond milk for cow's milk. If you are gluten-free, you can substitute gluten-free flour for regular flour. Try different alternatives to find what works best for you.

Meal plan with friends

Planning meals with a friend makes it more fun and less overwhelming. If you have a friend who follows a similar diet, consider planning meals together. This includes exchanging recipes, sharing meal prep tips, and cooking meals together. Don't be too hard on yourself

It's important to remember that following a special diet can be difficult and it's okay to make mistakes. If you make a mistake and eat something your diet doesn't allow, don't worry. Get back on track and continue your meal plan.

www.ingramcontent.com/pod-product-compliance
Lightning Source LLC
Chambersburg PA
CBHW061323250726